All you need to kn

Carnivore
Diet

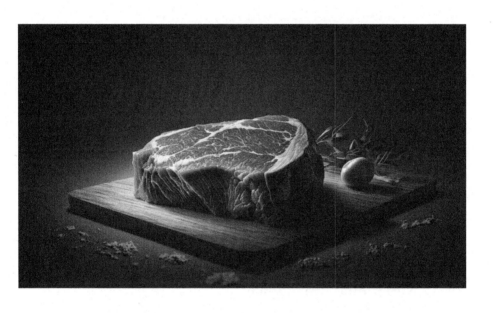

A Meat-Only Diet

Table of Contents

Introduction

Welcome to a journey all about the carnivore diet!

Have you ever heard of a diet where people eat only animal foods? It might sound surprising, but that's what the carnivore diet is all about. This way of eating focuses on meats and avoids foods from plants.

But why would someone choose to eat like this? Some people believe this diet is closer to how our ancient ancestors ate. Others feel it offers health benefits, like better energy or fewer health problems.

In this book, we'll explore everything you need to know about the carnivore diet. Whether you're curious, thinking of trying it, or just want to learn something new, we're here to help. We'll dive deep into its history, benefits, and even share some tasty recipes.

We've tried to keep things simple and easy to understand, especially for those who might be new to this topic or learning in a second language.

So, let's get started and discover the world of the carnivore diet together!

Background and Origins of the Carnivore Diet

The carnivore diet, as the name suggests, is about eating only animal-based foods. But where did this idea come from? Let's take a trip back in time.

Our Ancestors:
Long, long ago, our ancient ancestors, like the cavemen, ate what they could find. In cold places, plants were hard to find. So, they hunted animals for food. They ate everything from the animal - meat, fat, organs, and sometimes even bones.

Modern Times:
The idea of the carnivore diet in today's world isn't very old. Some people started trying it because they were curious. Others felt that modern diets with lots of sugar and processed foods were making them sick. They believed eating like our ancestors could make them feel better.

Health Reasons:
Over time, some people shared stories about how the carnivore diet helped their health problems. These stories made more people curious. They wondered if eating only animal foods could help them too.

The Internet Age:

With the growth of the internet, people began sharing their carnivore diet experiences online. Blogs, videos, and social media allowed people from different parts of the world to talk about this way of eating. This sharing made the diet more popular.

Science and Research:

In recent years, scientists and doctors have started studying the carnivore diet. They want to understand its benefits and risks better. Some studies suggest it might help with certain health problems. However, there's still much we don't know.

Conclusion

The carnivore diet has deep roots in our history. But its popularity in modern times is still growing. As we continue this book, we'll dive deeper into the details, benefits, and challenges of this unique way of eating.

Rise in Popularity and Modern Adaptations

The carnivore diet has become a big topic in recent years. But why? Let's explore how it became so talked about and the new ways people are trying it.

Health Success Stories:
Many people started trying the carnivore diet and then shared their stories online. Some said they lost weight. Others mentioned better energy, improved skin, or fewer health problems. These stories made many curious and eager to try it out.

Celebrities and Influencers:
When famous people talk, many listen. Some celebrities and online stars tried the carnivore diet and talked about it. This made more people interested in giving it a go.

The Internet and Social Media
Websites, blogs, YouTube videos, and social media posts about the carnivore diet spread the word fast. Online groups and forums let people ask questions, share tips, and support each other.

Books and Research:

Some doctors and experts wrote books about the carnivore diet. These books shared science, personal stories, and eating plans. They helped people understand the diet better.

Modern Twists:

Not everyone follows the carnivore diet in the same way. Some eat only beef, salt, and water. Others include different meats, eggs, and dairy. There are also versions like the "nose-to-tail" approach, where people eat all parts of the animal, including organs.

Challenges and Debates:

Not everyone agrees that the carnivore diet is good. Some worry about missing out on important nutrients from plants. Others question its long-term effects. These debates have made more people curious to learn and form their own opinions.

In conclusion, the carnivore diet's growth in popularity is because of many reasons. Personal stories, celebrity endorsements, and online sharing all played a part. Today, there are many ways people adapt and follow this diet. As we move forward in the book, we'll explore the pros, cons, and the science behind this eating style.

Chapter 1

Understanding the Basics

Before diving deep into the carnivore diet, it's important to know the simple stuff. What does "carnivore diet" really mean? How does it work? What foods are in, and which ones are out?

This section is like our starting line. Here, we'll explore the basic ideas of the carnivore diet. It's for everyone - whether you've heard a little about it or you're completely new to the topic. We'll break things down in easy-to-understand words and ideas.

So, if you're curious about the very heart of the carnivore diet, you're in the right place. Let's start our journey by getting to know its core principles!

Definition: What is the carnivore diet?

At its core, the carnivore diet is very simple. It's a way of eating where you mostly have foods that come from animals. This means meat, fish, and some animal products like eggs and certain dairy items. When you follow the carnivore diet, you usually don't eat plants. So, things like fruits, vegetables, grains, and nuts are not on the menu.

Imagine a plate full of steak, chicken, or fish. That's a typical meal on the carnivore diet.

Why do people choose this way of eating? Some believe it's more natural and closer to what our ancestors ate. Others feel better or see health benefits when they eat this way.

But, just like any diet, it's important to learn about it fully before trying. Everyone's body is different. What works well for one person might not be the best for another.

In the next sections, we'll dive deeper into the details. For now, just remember: the carnivore diet is all about eating animal foods and skipping the plants.

Core Principles of the Carnivore Diet

Animal-Based Foods
Meat: The heart of the carnivore diet is meat. This includes beef, pork, lamb, and poultry like chicken and turkey. Many people on this diet prefer fatty cuts of meat because they provide energy and make you feel full.

Fish
Fish is another main food on the carnivore diet. Both fatty fish (like salmon and mackerel) and lean fish (like cod and tilapia) are included.

Eggs
Eggs are highly nutritious and fit well into the carnivore way of eating. Both the white and the yolk are eaten.

Dairy
Some people on the carnivore diet eat dairy products like milk, cheese, and butter. However, not everyone includes dairy. It depends on how a person's body reacts to it. Some might find they feel better without dairy.

No Vegetables or Fruits

On many diets, vegetables and fruits are central. But on the carnivore diet, they are avoided. The idea is that some plants might have substances that aren't good for everyone's body.

No Grains

Foods like rice, wheat, and oats are not eaten on the carnivore diet. So, bread, pasta, and cereals are off the menu.

No Legumes

Beans, lentils, and peas are not eaten. These are plant foods that can be the main part of other diets but not on the carnivore one.

No Nuts or Seeds

Even though many consider them healthy, nuts and seeds are not part of the carnivore diet.

No Plant Oils

Instead of plant-based oils (like olive oil or sunflower oil), people on the carnivore diet might use animal fats for cooking. For example, butter or lard.

Variations of the Carnivore Diet

The carnivore diet has gained attention for its unique approach to nutrition. But, like many diets, there isn't just one way to follow it. Two main variations are the "strict carnivore" approach and the "hybrid" approach.

Strict Carnivore Approach

Only Animal Products: In the strictest form of the carnivore diet, only foods that come from animals are consumed. This means meat, fish, eggs, and, in some cases, dairy.

No Exceptions

People following this version avoid all plant-based foods, without any exceptions. That means no fruits, vegetables, nuts, seeds, legumes, or grains.

Water Over Other Drinks

In the strictest form, followers often drink only water. Some might also drink animal-based beverages, like bone broth.

Focus on Whole Foods

Processed meats (like sausages that have plant fillers) or products with added sugars and other non-animal ingredients are avoided.

Animal-Centric with Exceptions

While the focus remains on animal products, those following a hybrid approach allow certain plant foods into their diet. For instance, they might consume some vegetables, fruits, or even specific plant-based seasonings and spices.

Flexible with Dairy

Some people find that dairy products, especially in larger amounts, don't make them feel good. So, in the hybrid approach, they might limit or exclude dairy.

Inclusion of Beverages

Beyond just water, those on a hybrid approach might consume drinks like herbal teas, coffee, or other beverages that come from plants.

Conclusion

Each person's journey with the carnivore diet is unique. While some find that the strictest approach works best for their bodies and goals, others prefer the flexibility of a hybrid approach. It's essential for individuals to listen to their bodies and consult with health professionals. Adjusting the diet based on how one feels and the results one observes is key to finding a sustainable and healthful approach.

Chapter 2

Historical and Evolutionary Context

As we delve deeper into the carnivore diet, it's essential to root our understanding in the broader tapestry of human history and evolution. How did our ancestors eat? What did the diet of early humans look like? And how have these eating patterns influenced our biology and health?

This chapter will transport you back in time, exploring the dietary habits of ancient civilizations and tracing the evolutionary journey that has shaped our digestive systems and nutritional needs. By understanding the role of meat and plant foods in our history, we can gain a clearer perspective on the carnivore diet's place in the modern world. So, fasten your seatbelts and get ready for a fascinating journey through time and human evolution!

Ancestral Eating Habits

The Hunter-Gatherer Era

Before the advent of agriculture, our ancestors were hunter-gatherers, relying primarily on what they could hunt or gather for sustenance.

Meat Consumption: Hunting provided meat, a primary source of protein and fat. Early humans hunted a wide range of animals depending on their location and availability—from large mammals like mammoths and bison to smaller game and fish.

Plant-Based Foods: While hunting was crucial, gathering edible plants, fruits, seeds, and nuts also played a role in their diet. The percentage of plant-based foods in the diet varied based on the season, region, and availability.

Evolutionary Adaptations
The high reliance on meat led to certain evolutionary adaptations in humans.

Digestive System: Our stomachs produce a high concentration of hydrochloric acid, enabling us to break down animal proteins and fats effectively. Moreover, our small intestines are longer than those of herbivores, aiding in the absorption of nutrients from animal sources.

Brain Development: There's a theory that the nutrient-rich animal foods, especially fatty acids from fish and marrow, contributed significantly to the rapid expansion of the human brain.

Shift Towards Agriculture:
Around 10,000 years ago, with the Neolithic Revolution, humans began transitioning from a hunter-gatherer lifestyle to an agricultural one. This brought about a significant change in dietary patterns.

Increase in Plant Foods: As humans started cultivating crops, there was a rise in the consumption of grains, legumes, and eventually dairy. This led to a more carbohydrate-rich diet compared to the previous eras.

Domestication of Animals: While wild game was still hunted, the domestication of animals like cows, sheep, and chickens introduced consistent sources of meat, milk, and eggs.

Regional Variations
It's essential to understand that ancestral diets varied greatly depending on geography.

Arctic Regions: Indigenous groups like the Inuit primarily relied on marine mammals, fish, and other meats due to the scarcity of plant foods in their icy habitats.

Tropical Regions: Tribes living in more tropical climates had access to a wider variety of plant-based foods, such as fruits, tubers, and leafy greens, leading to a more balanced consumption of meat and plants.

Conclusion

Our ancestral eating habits were shaped by necessity, environment, and availability rather than choice. These early dietary patterns have influenced our genetic makeup and digestive capabilities. By understanding the diets of our ancestors, we can better comprehend why certain foods may be more natural and beneficial for our bodies to process.

Populations Known for Meat-Centric Diets

The Inuit of the Arctic

Diet Composition: Living in the icy terrains of Greenland, Canada, and Alaska, the Inuit primarily subsisted on marine mammals (like seals and whales), fish, and other meats as plant foods were scarce.

Adaptations: They developed unique metabolic adaptations to process the high fat content from marine animals. Interestingly, despite their fat-rich diet, they had a relatively low rate of heart diseases.

Cultural Importance: Meat was not only a dietary staple but also played a central role in their traditions, celebrations, and survival tactics.

The Maasai of East Africa

Diet Composition: This nomadic tribe's diet heavily featured cattle meat, milk, and blood. Plant foods were minimal in their consumption.

Health Implications: Despite their high animal fat intake, the Maasai displayed low cholesterol levels and were generally free from western chronic diseases.

Cultural Significance: Cattle were, and continue to be, a symbol of wealth and status among the Maasai, with their diet deeply rooted in their way of life and rituals.

The Mongols of Central Asia

Diet Composition: The Mongolian diet was mainly based on the livestock they herded, including sheep, cattle, camels, and horses. They consumed meat, dairy, and even horse blood.

Survival Strategy: Due to the harsh climates and their nomadic lifestyle, plant agriculture was limited. Hence, their diet was a pragmatic choice.

Historical Impact: The high-protein diet provided the energy and stamina required by the Mongol warriors during their vast conquests.

The Gauchos of South America

Diet Composition: These South American cowhands, especially from Argentina, were known for consuming vast amounts of beef, often cooked as 'asado' or barbecue.

Regional Influence: The vast grasslands, known as the Pampas, were perfect for cattle-raising, naturally skewing the diet of its inhabitants towards beef.

Cultural Heritage: The Gaucho's love for meat has left a lasting impact, with Argentina still known for its beef and barbecue culture.

Plains Indians of North America:

Diet Composition: Tribes like the Lakota Sioux primarily hunted bison, relying on it for meat, hides, and other essentials.

Holistic Usage: Every part of the bison was utilized, from meat for food, bones for tools, and hides for shelters and clothing.

Cultural and Spiritual Significance: The bison was central to their way of life and spirituality, symbolizing abundance and gratitude.

Conclusion

Throughout history, various populations around the world have thrived on meat-centric diets due to geographical, environmental, and cultural factors. Their health, vitality, and survival amidst challenging terrains and climates offer insights into the adaptability and resilience of the human body when consuming primarily animal-based foods.

Chapter 3

Benefits of the Carnivore Diet

In the vast tapestry of dietary choices, the carnivore diet stands out, often invoking intrigue and skepticism. After exploring its historical context and understanding its basic tenets, one might wonder: "Why adopt such a diet?" The answer lies in the myriad benefits that many of its adherents claim to experience. From heightened energy levels to improved mental clarity, the advantages span both physical and cognitive realms. While the carnivore diet isn't a one-size-fits-all solution, it offers a fascinating array of potential benefits that can transform one's health and well-being. In this chapter, we'll delve deep into these benefits, backed by personal anecdotes, emerging research, and a keen understanding of human physiology. Whether you're skeptical or curious, by the end of this chapter, you'll gain a comprehensive view of why the carnivore diet is more than just a modern dietary trend—it's a testament to the power of meat-centric nutrition.

Nutrient Density in Animal Foods

Nutrient density refers to the amount of essential nutrients packed in a given amount of food. When we consider nutrient density, animal foods, especially organ meats, are at the top of the list. They deliver a robust profile of vitamins, minerals, and other vital compounds often in more bioavailable forms compared to plant sources.

Vitamins

Vitamin B12
Exclusively found in animal products, B12 plays a crucial role in nerve function, red blood cell formation, and DNA synthesis. A deficiency can lead to anemia and neurological disorders.

Fat-soluble vitamins (A, D, E, and K)
Animal foods are rich in these vitamins, essential for various bodily functions. For instance, vitamin A from animal sources, known as retinol, is more easily utilized by our bodies than plant-based forms.

Vitamin B-Complex
Animal products, especially organ meats, are rich in B-vitamins like riboflavin, niacin, thiamin, pantothenic acid, pyridoxine, biotin, and folate. These are pivotal for energy metabolism, brain function, and DNA synthesis.

Minerals

Iron
Animal foods contain heme iron, which our bodies absorb more efficiently compared to the non-heme iron in plants.

Zinc
Crucial for immune function, protein synthesis, and DNA synthesis. Meat, especially red meat, is a top source of this mineral.

Selenium
An essential antioxidant that protects our cells. Fish and meats are prime sources.

Magnesium
Phosphorus, and Calcium: Abundantly found in fish, meat, and dairy.

Bioavailability

Animal-based nutrients often have a higher bioavailability, meaning our bodies can absorb and use them more efficiently. For example, the omega-3 fatty acids in fish are more readily available to us than the ALA form found in plants.

Essential Fatty Acids

Omega-3s

Found in fatty fish like salmon, mackerel, and sardines. These are crucial for brain health, inflammation control, and cardiovascular health.

Arachidonic Acid

This omega-6 fatty acid, found in meats, is vital for brain function and muscle growth.

Amino Acids

Animal proteins are complete proteins, meaning they provide all the essential amino acids our bodies need. This is pivotal for muscle growth, repair, and overall bodily functions.

Organ Meats – Nature's Multivitamin

Often referred to as "superfoods," organ meats like liver, heart, and kidney are packed with nutrients. For instance, beef liver is incredibly rich in copper, vitamin A, B-vitamins, and more.

Cholesterol - A misunderstood nutrient

Once demonized, cholesterol, found in animal foods, is vital for hormone production, vitamin D synthesis, and brain health. Our body produces its cholesterol, but dietary cholesterol has its roles, especially in hormone regulation.

Conclusion

While it's important to balance our diet and include a variety of foods, the nutrient density of animal products is undeniable. They offer a spectrum of essential nutrients in forms that our bodies can efficiently utilize. For those on a carnivore diet, it's essential to include a range of animal foods, especially organ meats, to harness the full array of nutrients.

Potential Advantages of the Carnivore Diet for Autoimmune Conditions

Autoimmune conditions arise when the body's immune system mistakenly targets and attacks its tissues. These conditions are multifactorial and can manifest in various ways, from rheumatoid arthritis and lupus to multiple sclerosis and celiac disease. Some proponents of the carnivore diet suggest that it may offer relief for autoimmune conditions. Let's explore the potential advantages:

Elimination of Potential Triggers
Gut Health: There's growing evidence that gut health plays a pivotal role in autoimmune conditions. Certain plant compounds, such as lectins and gluten, may increase gut permeability (often termed "leaky gut"), potentially leading to an autoimmune response. By removing these from the diet, the carnivore approach may help in reducing such triggers.

Reduction in Inflammation
Omega-6 to Omega-3 Ratio: Modern diets are often skewed toward omega-6 fatty acids, which, when consumed in excess, can promote inflammation. Animal foods, especially fatty fish, are rich in omega-3 fatty acids, known for their anti-inflammatory properties.

Saturated Fats: Contrary to previous beliefs, recent studies suggest that saturated fats, found abundantly in animal foods, might have anti-inflammatory effects, especially when plant-derived inflammatory compounds are removed.

Simplicity and the Removal of Variables

The carnivore diet, due to its restrictive nature, simplifies one's food intake. This makes it easier for individuals to pinpoint and remove foods that might trigger autoimmune flares.

Nutrient Density

Animal products, especially organ meats, are rich in nutrients like zinc, selenium, and vitamin D, which play crucial roles in immune function. Proper intake of these nutrients might support the body in regulating its immune response.

Enhanced Gut Health

Some individuals with autoimmune conditions report improved gut health on a carnivore diet. This could be due to:

Removal of Fiber: While fiber is often lauded for its gut health benefits, some people with autoimmune conditions, like Crohn's disease, find relief from symptoms when they reduce or eliminate fiber.

Increased Intake of Bone Broth: Many on the carnivore diet consume bone broth, which is rich in collagen and amino acids that can support gut lining health.

Mental Health and Autoimmunity

Stress and mental health can influence autoimmune flares. Some proponents of the carnivore diet report improved mood and mental clarity, potentially reducing triggers related to stress and anxiety.

Individual Variability and Personal Anecdotes

It's essential to note that many claims around the carnivore diet and autoimmunity are based on personal anecdotes. Some individuals report significant relief from autoimmune symptoms, while others might not see any change. Personal experiences can vary widely.

Caveats and Considerations:

While the carnivore diet might offer relief to some with autoimmune conditions, it's not a one-size-fits-all solution. Before making significant dietary changes:

Consultation: Always consult with healthcare professionals before adopting a restrictive diet, especially for those on medications or with severe conditions.

Nutritional Balance: Ensure the intake of a range of animal foods to cover the nutrient spectrum and avoid potential deficiencies.

Monitor Symptoms: Keep a close eye on autoimmune symptoms and general health markers to evaluate the diet's impact.

Conclusion

The carnivore diet's potential advantages for autoimmune conditions arise primarily from its elimination approach, nutrient density, and focus on animal-based foods. However, it's essential to approach with caution, ensure nutritional balance, and regularly consult with healthcare professionals to determine its efficacy and safety for individual circumstances.

Mental Clarity and Energy Levels on the Carnivore Diet

One of the often-touted benefits of the carnivore diet by its enthusiasts is enhanced mental clarity and boosted energy levels. Let's delve deep into understanding why some individuals might experience these effects when they consume an all-animal-based diet.

Stable Blood Sugar Levels

Reduced Carbohydrate Intake: A carnivore diet, devoid of carbohydrates, can lead to stable blood sugar levels. Avoiding the highs and lows associated with carbohydrate-rich meals might result in steadier energy throughout the day and less "brain fog."

Ketosis: In the absence of dietary carbohydrates, the body shifts to burning fat for fuel, producing ketones. Some believe that ketones, especially beta-hydroxybutyrate, are a more efficient brain fuel than glucose, potentially contributing to mental clarity.

Absence of Anti-Nutrients

Plant Compounds: Certain compounds in plants, like lectins and phytates, can interfere with nutrient absorption. By eliminating these, the carnivore diet may promote better nutrient utilization, potentially improving brain health and energy production.

Nutrient-Rich Diet

Brain Health: Animal foods are rich in essential nutrients like omega-3 fatty acids, choline, B12, and iron, which are critical for optimal brain function.

Mitochondrial Support: Nutrients like coenzyme Q10, present in meats, aid mitochondrial health. Since mitochondria are the "energy powerhouses" of our cells, their proper function is crucial for sustained energy and vitality.

Reduced Gut Inflammation

Brain-Gut Connection: An unhealthy gut can have a direct impact on brain health due to the gut-brain axis. Some individuals find relief from gut issues on the carnivore diet, which may translate to improved mental clarity.

Improved Sleep Patterns

Deep Sleep: Some anecdotal reports suggest better sleep quality on the carnivore diet. Better sleep can directly influence daytime energy levels and cognitive function.

Caveats and Individual Responses

Adaptation Phase: Initially, when transitioning to a carnivore diet, some people report fatigue and brain fog, often termed "keto flu." This is temporary and usually subsides as the body adapts to burning fat for fuel.

Electrolyte Imbalance: A diet change can lead to shifts in electrolyte balance, which might affect energy and cognition. It's crucial to ensure adequate intake of minerals like sodium, potassium, and magnesium.

The Importance of Personal Anecdotes

While not everyone might experience heightened mental clarity and energy on a carnivore diet, numerous personal accounts highlight these benefits. Such testimonies underscore the importance of individual variability in dietary responses.

Research and Understanding

It's worth noting that while anecdotal evidence is compelling, robust scientific research on the carnivore diet's effects on mental clarity and energy levels is still emerging. More studies are needed to validate and understand these claims fully.

Conclusion

The carnivore diet's potential to boost mental clarity and energy levels might stem from stable blood sugar levels, nutrient density, reduced gut inflammation, and other factors. However, individual responses can vary, and it's crucial to approach the diet with an open mind, attention to individual needs, and regular health monitoring.

Weight Loss and Body Composition Changes on the Carnivore Diet

The carnivore diet has attracted attention not just for its unique approach to nutrition, but also for its potential impact on weight loss and body composition. Let's dissect why and how this meat-centric diet might influence these factors.

Natural Caloric Reduction

Satiation and Satiety: Meat, being protein-rich, has a higher satiety index. This can make people feel full quicker and for longer periods, possibly leading to a spontaneous reduction in caloric intake.

Lack of Carbohydrates: Without the inclusion of carbohydrate-heavy foods, which can sometimes be calorie-dense, total caloric intake might decrease.

Enhanced Fat Burning

Shift to Ketosis: With the exclusion of carbs, the body may enter ketosis, a state where it burns fat for energy. This metabolic state is often linked with accelerated fat loss, especially when combined with a caloric deficit.

Stabilized Insulin Levels: Lower insulin levels, due to a lack of dietary carbohydrates, can facilitate fat burning by reducing insulin resistance and improving metabolic health.

Muscle Preservation

High Protein Intake: A diet abundant in protein is critical for muscle preservation, especially when in a caloric deficit. The carnivore diet, being predominantly protein-rich, can ensure muscle retention during weight loss.

Essential Amino Acids: Animal foods provide all the essential amino acids in the right ratios, supporting muscle synthesis and repair.

Reduced Water Retention

Loss of Glycogen: Carbohydrates are stored as glycogen in the muscles and liver. Each gram of glycogen is bound to approximately 3-4 grams of water. A reduction in dietary carbs leads to a loss of glycogen stores, and consequently, water weight. This can result in immediate weight loss, especially during the initial phase of the diet.

Lowered Insulin: Insulin can cause the kidneys to retain sodium and water. Reduced insulin levels on a carnivore diet can promote diuresis (increased urine production), leading to a loss of excess water weight.

Hormonal Benefits

Leptin and Ghrelin: The carnivore diet may influence hormones that regulate hunger and satiety, leading to reduced food intake and potential weight loss.

Improved Thyroid Function: While research is still nascent, some anecdotal reports suggest better thyroid health on a carnivore diet, which can influence metabolism and weight.

Individual Variability:

Metabolic Rate: Individual metabolic rates can vary. While some might experience rapid weight loss, others might notice slower changes or even weight maintenance.

Activity Levels: The benefits on weight and body composition can be further influenced by one's level of physical activity.

Potential Pitfalls

Overconsumption: Just because the diet is low in carbs doesn't mean one can eat unlimited amounts of meat without considering calorie intake. Overeating can offset any potential weight loss benefits.

Micronutrient Balance: While focusing on macronutrients, it's essential not to overlook vitamins and minerals that influence metabolism and overall health.

Research and Understanding

Current understanding is based on a mix of scientific research, anecdotal evidence, and expert opinion. It's essential to remember that in-depth, long-term research specifically on the carnivore diet's impact on weight and body composition is still in its early stages.

Conclusion

The carnivore diet presents a unique approach to weight loss and body composition, potentially offering benefits like enhanced fat burning, muscle preservation, and reduced water retention. Individual experiences will vary, and it's vital to approach this dietary strategy with proper knowledge, monitoring, and expert guidance.

Chapter 4

Common Concerns and Criticisms of the Carnivore Diet

When new dietary patterns emerge, they often come with a mix of intrigue, advocacy, doubt, and skepticism. The carnivore diet, with its radical departure from conventional dietary advice, is no exception. While its proponents sing praises of its numerous potential benefits, a chorus of critics raises genuine concerns. In this section, we will dive deep into the most common apprehensions and critiques related to the carnivore diet, seeking to separate myth from fact, and to provide a balanced view for those contemplating this nutritional approach.

Nutrient Deficiencies in the Carnivore Diet

Vitamin C

The General Concern
The carnivore diet largely excludes fruits and vegetables, which are primary sources of Vitamin C for many. This has led to concerns that following a strictly animal-based diet might lead to a deficiency in this essential vitamin.

The Carnivore Perspective
Advocates of the carnivore diet argue that the requirement for Vitamin C decreases when one consumes fewer carbohydrates. Additionally, they point out that fresh meat, especially organ meats like liver, contains small amounts of Vitamin C, which might be sufficient in the absence of high carbohydrate intake. Historically, sailors and explorers prevented scurvy (a disease caused by Vitamin C deficiency) with fresh meat when fruits were unavailable.

What the Science Says
It's true that organ meats provide Vitamin C, but the quantities are significantly lower than in fruits and vegetables. While reduced carbohydrate intake might decrease the need for Vitamin C, the long-term implications of this on overall health remain understudied.

Fiber

The General Concern

Dietary fiber, predominantly found in plant-based foods, aids digestion, promotes gut health, and has been linked to reduced risks of various diseases, including colon cancer and cardiovascular diseases. A diet devoid of plant sources might lead to a fiber deficiency, raising concerns about digestive health and disease risks.

The Carnivore Perspective

Proponents argue that fiber is not essential for human health. They suggest that the human digestive system can function optimally without fiber, pointing out that many people on the carnivore diet report fewer digestive issues, such as bloating and irregular bowel movements.

What the Science Says

While it's true that some people may find relief from specific digestive issues when eliminating fibrous foods, the broader health benefits of dietary fiber, especially for gut microbiota and colon health, are well-established in scientific literature. It's also worth noting that everyone's body reacts differently; some may do well without fiber, while others may experience constipation or other issues.

Other Potential Nutrient Concerns

There are other nutrients primarily found in plants, such as certain B vitamins, magnesium, and potassium, which could be of concern on a strict carnivore diet. However, many of these nutrients are also present in animal foods, especially in organ meats. For instance, liver is rich in various nutrients and can provide many of the vitamins and minerals missing from muscle meat. Still, relying on a very limited range of foods can always introduce potential nutrient gaps.

Conclusion

While the carnivore diet offers certain benefits, potential nutrient deficiencies are a legitimate concern. Those interested in pursuing this diet should be well-informed and consider periodic health check-ups to ensure they are not developing any deficiencies.

Long-Term Sustainability and Potential Risks

Long-Term Sustainability

The General Concern

Many nutritionists and health experts question whether the carnivore diet can be sustained in the long run. A diet based solely on animal products lacks variety, and sticking to it may become monotonous for many, leading to potential "diet fatigue."

The Carnivore Perspective

Devotees of the diet argue that its simplicity is its strength. By eliminating the need to choose from a vast array of foods, decision-making is streamlined, potentially making it easier to stick to the diet. They also argue that the significant benefits they experience, such as increased energy and mental clarity, motivate them to continue.

What the Science Says

Dietary variety is often linked to better overall nutrient intake and long-term adherence to dietary changes. While some might find the carnivore diet's simplicity appealing, others may struggle with the lack of variety, potentially leading to nutrient deficiencies or a return to previous eating habits.

Potential Risks

Heart Health

The General Concern

A diet high in red and processed meats has been linked to an increased risk of heart diseases due to high levels of saturated fats and cholesterol.

The Carnivore Perspective

Proponents argue that recent research challenges the belief that saturated fats are detrimental to heart health. They also claim that the diet can improve heart health markers, such as reducing triglycerides and increasing HDL ("good") cholesterol.

What the Science Says

While some recent studies question the link between saturated fats and heart disease, the consensus remains that a diet rich in unsaturated fats and low in saturated fats is beneficial for heart health.

Bone Health

The General Concern

Without dairy or fortified plant-based sources, there might be a lack of calcium in the diet, potentially risking bone health.

The Carnivore Perspective

Many carnivore dieters include bone broths and small fish, which are rich in calcium. They argue that these sources, combined with vitamin D from the diet, can support bone health.

What the Science Says

Bone health is influenced by multiple nutrients, including calcium, vitamin D, magnesium, and phosphorus. While certain animal foods can provide these nutrients, the absence of diverse sources might pose risks in the long run.

Kidney Function

The General Concern

High protein diets can be challenging for the kidneys and may exacerbate issues in those with existing kidney conditions.

The Carnivore Perspective

The diet is often high in fat, not just protein, and as such, the protein content isn't necessarily excessive. Additionally, for those with healthy kidneys, a higher protein intake is generally considered safe.

What the Science Says

For individuals with healthy kidneys, a high protein intake doesn't seem to pose significant risks. However, those with kidney issues or at risk should consult with healthcare professionals before making drastic dietary changes.

Conclusion

While the carnivore diet presents potential benefits, the long-term sustainability and risks are valid concerns. It's essential for individuals to weigh the pros and cons, be well-informed, and consider periodic health assessments if they choose to adopt this dietary approach.

Ethical and Environmental Considerations of the Carnivore Diet

Ethical Considerations

The General Concern
Adopting a diet solely based on animal products raises questions about animal welfare. Factory farming practices are known for their questionable treatment of animals and are the primary source of meat for many.

The Carnivore Perspective
Many adherents of the carnivore diet are aware of these concerns and opt for grass-fed, pasture-raised, or wild-caught sources. They argue that this not only provides a higher nutrient profile but also supports more ethical treatment of animals.

What the Science and Ethics Say
Grass-fed and pasture-raised animal farming methods are generally considered more ethical due to better living conditions for the animals. However, ethical considerations can be subjective and might also involve concerns about taking animal life for food when alternatives are available.

Environmental Considerations

Resource Consumption

The General Concern
Producing meat, especially beef, requires significant amounts of water, land, and feed compared to plant-based foods.

The Carnivore Perspective
Some proponents argue that regenerative agriculture, which involves practices like rotational grazing, can mitigate these impacts, turning cattle farming into a more sustainable practice that can even help sequester carbon.

What the Science Says
Regenerative agriculture practices show promise in reducing the environmental footprint of animal farming. However, on a global scale, plant-based foods still generally use fewer resources than animal-based foods.

Greenhouse Gas Emissions

The General Concern
Animal agriculture, particularly ruminants like cows, produces significant amounts of methane, a potent greenhouse gas.

The Carnivore Perspective
Again, the argument for regenerative agriculture comes into play. Proponents suggest that well-managed pastures can sequester enough carbon to offset the methane produced by ruminants.

What the Science Says
While well-managed pastures can indeed sequester carbon, the extent to which this can offset methane emissions from ruminants is a topic of ongoing research. Current consensus is that reducing meat consumption is a beneficial strategy for lowering greenhouse gas emissions.

Biodiversity

The General Concern
Large-scale animal farming can lead to deforestation and habitat destruction, endangering biodiversity.

The Carnivore Perspective

Some argue that sustainable hunting and fishing practices, as well as supporting small-scale, local farms, can reduce these impacts.

What the Science Says

Sustainable hunting, fishing, and local farming do have a smaller ecological footprint. However, the scalability of these practices to meet global meat demand without impacting biodiversity remains uncertain.

Conclusion

While the carnivore diet presents potential health benefits for some individuals, it comes with significant ethical and environmental considerations. Potential adopters should be aware of these issues and consider sourcing methods and their broader impact when making dietary choices.

Chapter 5

Nutritional Breakdown

When embarking on any dietary journey, it's essential to have a clear understanding of the nutrients you'll be consuming. With the carnivore diet, this becomes even more crucial, given its unique emphasis on animal-based foods. But what exactly are the nutritional components of this diet? Are all meats the same in terms of nutrition? What about organ meats, seafood, and other animal-derived products?

In this chapter, we will delve deep into the nutrient profile of a carnivorous diet. We'll explore the vitamins, minerals, proteins, fats, and other compounds present in various animal foods. We aim to provide you with a comprehensive view, ensuring you make informed decisions and maximize the health benefits while following the carnivore lifestyle. Whether you're a seasoned carnivore dieter or someone just beginning to explore this pathway, this chapter will offer valuable insights into the building blocks of the foods central to this diet.

Essential Nutrients in a Carnivore Diet

A carnivore diet, with its emphasis on animal products, offers a rich source of several essential nutrients. These nutrients play vital roles in maintaining optimal bodily functions, supporting growth, and ensuring overall health. Let's delve into some of the primary nutrients prevalent in this diet:

Protein

Significance: Proteins are the building blocks of the body. They support muscle growth, repair tissues, and are crucial for enzyme and hormone production.

Sources: All animal meats, including beef, chicken, fish, and pork, are rich sources of high-quality, complete proteins, meaning they provide all the essential amino acids the body requires.

Fats

Significance: Fats are a primary energy source, support cell growth, and are necessary for the absorption of certain vitamins.

Sources: Animal meats, especially fatty cuts, and certain seafood, like salmon, provide both saturated and unsaturated fats. Organ meats and egg yolks also contribute beneficial fats like omega-3 fatty acids.

Vitamin B12

Significance: Vital for nerve function, the formation of red blood cells, and DNA synthesis.

Sources: Found exclusively in animal products, including meat, fish, poultry, and eggs.

Iron

Significance: Essential for oxygen transportation in the blood and muscle function.

Sources: Red meats, especially organ meats like liver, are particularly high in heme iron, which is more efficiently absorbed by the body compared to plant-based iron sources.

Zinc

Significance: Supports the immune system, wound healing, and DNA synthesis.

Sources: Red meats, seafood (especially oysters), and poultry.

Creatine

Significance: Stored in muscles, it helps produce energy during high-intensity, short-duration exercises.

Sources: Red meat, pork, poultry, and fish.

Carnosine

Significance: A compound that can reduce oxidative stress and inflammation in the body.

Sources: Found in significant amounts in beef, poultry, and pork.

Taurine

Significance: An amino acid that supports bile salt formation, antioxidant defenses, and may benefit heart health.

Sources: Meat and fish, especially in the heart and brain tissues.

Vitamin D

Significance: Essential for bone health, immune function, and inflammation control.

Sources: Fatty fish, like salmon and mackerel, and fortified animal products.

Cholesterol

Significance: Despite its controversial reputation, cholesterol is essential for the body, aiding in the synthesis of vitamin D, hormones, and bile acids.

Sources: Egg yolks, organ meats, and shellfish.

Omega-3 Fatty Acids

Significance: Support heart health, brain function, and possess anti-inflammatory properties.

Sources: Fatty fish, like salmon and sardines, and certain meats, such as grass-fed beef.

Vitamin K2

Significance: Works in conjunction with calcium and vitamin D to maintain bone and heart health.

Sources: Egg yolks, high-fat dairy products, and organ meats.

While a carnivore diet can provide many of the essential nutrients the body requires, it's important to diversify one's meat intake. Incorporating a range of animal products, from muscle meats to organ meats and seafood, can help ensure a comprehensive nutrient profile.

Sourcing Quality Meats: Grass-fed vs. Grain-fed, Wild-caught, and More

Meat quality plays a pivotal role in the nutrient profile and overall benefits one can reap from a carnivore diet. The method of farming, the diet of the animals, and the conditions they are raised in can significantly influence the nutritional value and ethical considerations of the meats consumed. Let's delve into the different sources of meat and their respective benefits and considerations:

Grass-fed vs. Grain-fed Meat

Grass-fed

Nutritional Benefits: Tends to be leaner and contains a healthier fat profile, often having higher levels of omega-3 fatty acids, antioxidants like vitamin E, and increased amounts of Vitamin K2.

Environmental & Ethical Benefits: Grass-fed animals often graze in open pastures, leading to better animal welfare. Their farming can also be more sustainable, contributing to soil health.

Taste & Texture: Many people find that grass-fed meat has a more robust, earthy flavor compared to grain-fed counterparts.

Grain-fed

Nutritional Profile: Typically contains more overall fat, but less of the beneficial omega-3 fatty acids and other nutrients prevalent in grass-fed varieties.

Economic Considerations: Grain-fed meats are generally less expensive and more widely available in most grocery stores. Environmental Concerns: The mass production of grain-fed animals can have significant environmental impacts, including deforestation and higher greenhouse gas emissions.

Wild-caught vs. Farm-raised Seafood

Wild-caught

Nutritional Benefits: Wild fish tend to have a more favorable fatty acid profile, with higher omega-3s and fewer omega-6s. They also are less likely to have contaminants like antibiotics or pesticides.

Taste & Texture: Offers a more natural and often more pronounced flavor, with a firmer texture.

Environmental Considerations: Overfishing is a significant concern, making it essential to choose species that are sustainably sourced.

Farm-raised

Nutritional Differences: Might contain more omega-6 fatty acids and likely harmful substances due to farming conditions.

Economic Factors: Often less expensive than wild-caught and can be farmed sustainably with the right practices.

Environmental Benefits and Concerns: Aquaculture can reduce the strain on overfished populations but can also lead to issues like water pollution if not managed responsibly. Free-range Poultry vs. Conventionally Raised:

Free-range

Nutritional Benefits: Often contains a better fat profile and fewer antibiotics or growth hormones.

Ethical Considerations: Birds typically have more freedom to roam, leading to better living conditions.

Conventionally Raised

Economic Considerations: More widely available and often less expensive.

Nutritional and Ethical Concerns: These birds often live in crowded conditions and may have been given antibiotics or growth hormones.

Organic vs. Non-organic Meats

Organic

Nutritional & Health Benefits: Organic meats are free from antibiotics, growth hormones, and genetically modified organisms. They might also have a slightly better nutrient profile.

Environmental Benefits: Organic farming practices often prioritize sustainability and eco-friendliness.
Non-organic:

Economic Factors: Typically less expensive than organic meats.

Potential Concerns: Exposure to pesticides, antibiotics, and other chemicals is a significant concern for many consumers.

Organ Meats and Their Importance

Often referred to as "nature's multivitamins", organ meats, or offal, are the internal organs and entrails of animals. They have been consumed by various cultures throughout history and are considered delicacies in many parts of the world. When following a carnivore diet, integrating organ meats can be a game-changer for several reasons:

Nutrient Density

Vitamins & Minerals: Organ meats are some of the most nutrient-dense foods on the planet. Liver, for instance, is a rich source of vitamin A, iron, and B vitamins. Kidneys are loaded with selenium and B12. Heart contains CoQ10, a nutrient beneficial for heart health.

Complete Proteins: They offer all the essential amino acids the body needs, making them a valuable protein source, especially for those avoiding plant-based foods.

Bioavailability

The nutrients in organ meats are in forms that the body can easily absorb. For example, the iron in organ meats is heme iron, which the body absorbs more efficiently than the non-heme iron found in plant foods.

Budget-Friendly Nutrition

Due to their lesser demand in many Western cultures, organ meats tend to be less expensive than muscle meats. This makes them an economical way to enrich one's diet with high-quality nutrients.

Historical and Ancestral Relevance

Traditional societies often prioritized the consumption of organ meats over muscle meats due to their superior nutritional profile. They recognized the health benefits long before modern nutrition science validated their choices.

Diversity in Diet

Different organ meats have distinct flavors and textures, adding variety to a carnivorous diet. From the creaminess of liver pâté to the chewiness of heart slices, they can be prepared in various ways to suit different palates.

Satiety and Gut Health

Nutrients like glycine found in organ meats (especially in tripe and other connective tissues) can support gut health and overall inflammation in the body. Also, the nutrient density can lead to increased feelings of fullness, assisting in appetite regulation.

Ethical Considerations

Eating the entire animal, including its organs, follows the "nose-to-tail" approach, minimizing waste and honoring the animal. Organ meats are nutritionally rich, offering vital nutrients that muscle meats might miss. They're essential for a balanced carnivore diet.

Chapter 6

Transitioning to a Carnivore Diet

Embarking on a new dietary journey can often be akin to setting sail into uncharted waters. The carnivore diet, with its unique emphasis on animal products and elimination of plant-based foods, certainly represents a departure from conventional dietary norms for many. As you stand on the precipice of this dietary transition, questions and uncertainties might flood your mind: How will your body react? What can you expect in the initial days? And most importantly, how can you make this transition smooth and sustainable?

This chapter aims to be your guiding compass, offering insights and strategies to navigate this dietary shift with confidence. We'll delve into the initial phases, the potential challenges you might face, and provide practical tips to ease into a carnivore lifestyle. Whether you're driven by curiosity, health reasons, or a quest for personal optimization, understanding the nuances of this transition can be pivotal for a successful and enjoyable carnivore journey.

So, buckle up and get ready, as we guide you step by step through the transformative process of embracing a carnivore diet.

Gradual vs. Immediate Transitions

When embracing a new diet, especially one as distinct as the carnivore diet, individuals often ponder the best approach: Should they dive in headfirst or wade in slowly? Both methods come with their own set of advantages and challenges. Let's explore them in depth:

Gradual Transition

Advantages

Ease into Change: A slow shift allows your body and mind to adapt without overwhelming shock. It can help mitigate adverse reactions as the digestive system slowly adjusts to the new food intake.

Psychological Comfort: For many, the idea of abruptly giving up a vast range of foods can be daunting. Gradual change can alleviate some of this anxiety, providing a comfort zone while you're still making progress.

Flexibility: This approach gives you time to research, understand, and figure out the best sources for quality meats and animal products.

Challenges

Delayed Benefits: Since you're not fully adopting the carnivore diet immediately, it might take longer to start observing its potential benefits.

Temptations: A slower shift means that non-carnivore foods are still part of your diet for a while, which could lead to temptations or inconsistency in sticking to the plan.

Immediate Transition

Advantages

Rapid Results: By jumping straight into the carnivore diet, you might start experiencing its benefits sooner, from increased energy levels to potential improvements in specific health markers.

Clear Boundaries: An immediate shift offers clear dietary guidelines. There's less room for ambiguity about what's allowed and what isn't, which can be helpful for some individuals.

Detox and Adaptation: While it might be challenging, plunging in can allow your body to detox from certain foods and adapt to its new fuel source more swiftly.

Challenges

Initial Discomfort: An abrupt change in diet might lead to temporary side effects, such as digestive discomfort, fatigue, or mood swings, commonly referred to as "keto flu" when transitioning to low-carb diets.

Mental Challenge: A sudden elimination of all plant-based foods can be mentally challenging, especially if you've never tried restrictive diets before.

Preparation: You'll need to be well-prepared, ensuring you have the right foods at hand and a clear understanding of the diet's principles from day one.

Conclusion

The choice between a gradual or immediate transition largely depends on individual preferences, current health status, and personal goals. Some might find solace in the slow and steady approach, while others may thrive on the immediate challenge. It's crucial to listen to your body, seek guidance when needed, and adjust the course as you deem fit. Whatever path you choose, the key lies in commitment and understanding the reasons behind your choice.

Managing Initial Side Effects of the Carnivore Diet

Transitioning to a diet based solely or mainly on animal products is a significant shift for most people. During this period of adjustment, you might experience several temporary side effects. Understanding and preparing for these can make the process smoother.

Digestive Changes

Symptoms: Changes in bowel habits, bloating, gas, or indigestion.

Management:

- Stay hydrated to help digestion.
- Opt for leaner cuts initially and slowly introduce fattier meats as your digestion improves.
- Consider digestive enzymes or bone broth for gut health.

"Carnivore Flu"

Symptoms: Fatigue, dizziness, headaches, and irritability, similar to the "keto flu."

Management:

- Ensure adequate electrolyte intake, especially sodium, potassium, and magnesium.
- Drink plenty of water.
- Rest when needed and avoid heavy activities in the early days.

Energy Slumps

Symptoms: Feeling lethargic or experiencing decreased energy levels.

Management:
- Consume adequate calories. Remember, you might need more food than you think.
- Break meals into smaller portions spread throughout the day.
- Ensure a balance of protein and fats for sustained energy.

Sleep Disruptions

Symptoms: Trouble falling asleep or waking up frequently.

Management:
- Limit caffeine intake, especially in the afternoon and evening.
- Establish a consistent sleep routine.
- Ensure your room is dark, quiet, and cool.

Cravings

Symptoms: Intense desire for foods, especially carbohydrates or sugars.

Management:

- Consume satiating meals with adequate fat and protein.
- Find carnivore-friendly "snack" options for moments of intense cravings.
- Distract yourself with activities or tasks to divert attention from cravings.

Changes in Muscle Function

Symptoms: Muscle cramps or twitches.

Management:

- Again, ensure you're getting enough electrolytes in your diet.
- Gentle stretches and movement can help alleviate cramps.
- Consider magnesium supplements if the problem persists.

It's important to note that while these side effects are common, they don't occur for everyone and often resolve after a few days or weeks. It's always essential to listen to your body. If severe issues arise or persist, it's advisable to consult with a healthcare professional. Remember, everyone's experience is unique, and personal adjustments might be needed based on individual responses to the diet.

Supplements to Consider During Carnivore Diet Transition

Electrolytes

Why: As your body adapts to consuming fewer carbohydrates, there might be an initial diuresis where you excrete more water and electrolytes.

What to consider: Sodium, potassium, and magnesium are the primary electrolytes to focus on.

Digestive Enzymes

Why: To aid digestion, especially if you're consuming more fats and proteins than you're used to.

What to consider: Look for a broad-spectrum enzyme supplement that includes lipase (for fat digestion) and protease (for protein digestion).

Omega-3 Fatty Acids

Why: While the carnivore diet can be rich in Omega-3s, especially if you consume fatty fish, supplementing can ensure optimal levels.

What to consider: Fish oil or krill oil supplements.

Vitamin D

Why: If you're not consuming fatty fish regularly or getting adequate sun exposure, you might lack this essential vitamin.

What to consider: Vitamin D3 supplements.

Magnesium

Why: Helps in muscle function and can alleviate muscle cramps or twitches.

What to consider: Magnesium citrate or magnesium glycinate.

Bone Broth

Why: Contains essential minerals and can help support gut health during the transition.

What to consider: High-quality bone broth, either homemade or store-bought.

Vitamin C

Why: While fresh meat contains vitamin C, those who are concerned about intake might consider a supplement.

What to consider: A low-dose vitamin C supplement.

Taurine

Why: This amino acid supports heart and brain health and might be beneficial, especially if not consuming organ meats.

What to consider: Taurine supplement.

It's essential to use supplements as tools, not crutches. Before starting any supplement regimen, always consult with a healthcare professional. As you progress on the carnivore diet, you may find that you need fewer supplements or different ones based on your personal needs and food choices. Listening to your body and being adaptable is key.

Chapter 7

Sample Meal Plans and Recipes

Embracing the carnivore diet doesn't mean diving into a world of monotony. In fact, it opens the doors to a rich culinary journey where the spotlight is on the pure, authentic flavors of animal-based foods. Whether you're an experienced chef or someone who's more comfortable with basic cooking, this chapter promises to guide you through a variety of delectable meals tailored for the carnivore enthusiast. From simple yet hearty breakfasts to sumptuous dinners, we'll walk you through detailed meal plans and recipes that not only nourish the body but also delight the palate. Let's embark on this flavorful adventure and bring the essence of the carnivore diet to your table!

Breakfast Ideas 🍳

Classic Steak and Eggs

A juicy ribeye paired with sunny-side-up eggs. Seasoned lightly with salt.

Bacon-Wrapped Sausages

Sausages wrapped in thick-cut bacon strips and pan-fried until crispy.

Salmon Roe with Butter

Fresh salmon roe served with slices of salted butter on the side.

Bone Broth

A warm cup of bone broth made from slow-cooked beef or chicken bones, perfect to kickstart the metabolism.

Lunch Ideas

Roast Chicken

A whole roasted chicken seasoned with just salt. Can be paired with chicken liver pate for added nutrition.

Tuna Steak

A thick-cut tuna steak seared on each side for a tender inside and a slightly crispy exterior.

Beef Liver Stir-fry

Thinly sliced beef liver stir-fried in beef tallow with salt to taste.

Pork Chops

Juicy pork chops grilled to perfection. Can be eaten with a side of bone marrow for added flavor and nutrition.

Dinner Ideas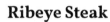

Ribeye Steak

A generously sized ribeye steak grilled or pan-seared with beef tallow or butter.

Lamb Kebabs

Skewered pieces of lamb marinated in animal fat and grilled until slightly charred.

Butter Poached Lobster Tails

Lobster tails poached gently in melted butter, showcasing the richness of the seafood.

Duck Confit

Duck legs slowly cooked in their own fat until they're incredibly tender on the inside and have a crisp skin on the outside.

Snack Ideas

Pork Rinds
Crispy, salted pork skins, either homemade or store-bought without any added flavorings.

Beef Jerky
Thin strips of beef dried and seasoned with just salt.

Bone Marrow
Roasted bones with the marrow scooped out and eaten directly or spread on meat slices.

Hard Cheeses (for those allowing dairy)
Varieties like Parmesan or aged cheddar, enjoyed in small amounts.

Remember, while these meal ideas embrace the carnivore spirit, it's essential to listen to your body and adjust based on personal preferences and nutritional needs. Experiment with various cuts and types of meats to keep the diet interesting and enjoyable.

Cooking techniques for various meats

Beef

Grilling
Best for steaks like ribeye, sirloin, and filet mignon. This method imparts a smoky flavor and sears the outside, locking in juices. Season simply with salt, and cook over high heat for a short duration for medium-rare to medium doneness.

Roasting
Ideal for larger cuts like prime rib or a whole beef tenderloin. Roasting in an oven at a consistent temperature ensures even cooking.

Braising
Perfect for tougher cuts like chuck, brisket, or short ribs. Slow-cooking in liquid breaks down the tough fibers, resulting in tender, flavorful meat.

Pan-searing
For steaks and beef slices. Creates a delicious crust on the meat's exterior while keeping the inside juicy.

Poultry (Chicken, Turkey, Duck)

Roasting

This method cooks the bird evenly, yielding crispy skin. Season the bird inside and out, truss it, and roast in an oven.

Grilling

Ideal for chicken breasts, thighs, or wings. Marinate or season as desired, and grill over medium heat.

Poaching

Great for chicken breasts. Gently simmering in water or broth retains moisture and ensures tender meat.

Braising

Best for duck legs or chicken thighs. The slow-cooking in liquid ensures a rich flavor and melt-in-the-mouth texture.

Pork

Grilling

Suitable for pork chops or tenderloin. Season and grill over medium-high heat.

Roasting

Ideal for pork loins or a whole ham. Season and roast in an oven.

Braising

Best for pork belly or shoulder. This method ensures flavorful, fork-tender meat.

Pan-frying

For thin pork cutlets or bacon strips. This method crisps the meat and locks in flavor.

Fish and Seafood

Grilling

Best for meaty fish like salmon, tuna, or swordfish steaks. Ensure the grill is very hot to prevent sticking.

Poaching

Suitable for delicate fish like cod or sole. Simmering in a flavorful liquid ensures moist and flaky fish.

Pan-searing

Ideal for skin-on fish fillets. The method creates a crispy skin and tender interior.

Steaming

Best for shellfish like mussels, clams, or crab. This gentle method retains the natural flavors.

Organ Meats

Pan-frying

Liver, kidney, or heart can be thinly sliced, seasoned, and quickly pan-fried in butter or animal fat.

Braising

Tougher organs like tongue or heart benefit from slow-cooking in flavorful liquid.

When cooking meats, especially for a carnivore diet, it's essential to:

- Avoid charring or overcooking, which can produce harmful compounds.
- Use quality fats like butter, tallow, or ghee.
- Ensure safe handling and thorough cooking to avoid foodborne illnesses.
- Experimenting with these techniques can provide a variety of flavors and textures, making the carnivore diet both enjoyable and gastronomically fulfilling.

Incorporating Organ Meats and Less Common Animal Products

The Importance of Organ Meats

Organ meats, often referred to as "offal", are some of the most nutrient-dense foods available. They provide essential vitamins, minerals, and amino acids that may be less abundant in muscle meats.

Common Organ Meats and Their Benefits

Liver: Often called nature's multivitamin, liver is a powerhouse of nutrients. It is rich in vitamin A, B vitamins (especially B12 and folate), iron, choline, and copper. Beef, chicken, and lamb liver are popular choices.

Heart: A rich source of coenzyme Q10 (CoQ10), which is vital for heart health. It's also high in B vitamins, iron, and zinc.

Kidney: High in selenium, iron, and B12. It also contains anti-inflammatory omega-3 fatty acids.

Tongue: Though not technically an organ, it's a great source of fat, iron, zinc, choline, and vitamin B12.

Brain: Rich in omega-3 fatty acids, especially DHA, which is crucial for brain health. It also contains important fat-soluble vitamins and cholesterol.

Less Common Animal Products and Their Benefits

Bone Marrow: A source of beneficial fats, collagen, and essential nutrients like vitamin B12, vitamin K2, and minerals such as zinc, manganese, and iron.

Bone Broth: Made by simmering bones over a long period, it's rich in collagen, amino acids like glycine, and minerals like calcium and phosphorus.

Fish Roe (Fish Eggs): Particularly rich in omega-3 fatty acids, vitamin D, and other fat-soluble vitamins.

Feet, Tails, and Hooves: When simmered, these parts release gelatin and collagen, making them great for gut health.

Tips for Incorporating Organ Meats

Start Slowly: For those unfamiliar with the taste, it's advisable to start with milder organs like liver or heart. Gradually introduce others over time.

Mix with Muscle Meats: Blend organ meats with regular meats. For instance, mix ground liver with ground beef for burgers.

Experiment with Recipes: Pâtés, sausages, and stews can mask the strong flavors of some organs.

Source High-Quality Organ Meats: Ensure that the organs come from animals raised in good conditions, preferably grass-fed or pasture-raised.

Frequency: Aim to include organ meats 1-3 times a week to diversify nutrient intake.

Embracing organ meats and other lesser-known animal products can significantly enhance the nutrient density of a carnivore diet. With time and experimentation, many find these once unfamiliar foods to become enjoyable staples in their meals.

Chapter 8

Personal Testimonies and Case Studies

Every journey is unique, and in the realm of diets and lifestyle changes, personal experiences often speak louder than generalized advice or statistical evidence. The carnivore diet, while supported by numerous scientific studies, truly comes to life when we delve into the real stories of individuals who've walked the path, experienced the challenges, and reaped the benefits. In this chapter, we'll explore authentic testimonies and detailed case studies, shedding light on the transformative power of an all-meat diet from diverse perspectives. From overcoming chronic illnesses to achieving unprecedented levels of fitness and well-being, these stories will inspire, inform, and perhaps, resonate with your own aspirations.

Real-life Success Stories

Every transformative journey is marked by stories of success, perseverance, and learning. The carnivore diet, being no exception, boasts a tapestry of real-life experiences. Let's dive into a few such stories:

Alexandra's Triumph over Chronic Fatigue

Background: For over a decade, Alexandra battled chronic fatigue syndrome. Daily tasks felt mountainous, and she couldn't recall a day without feeling drained.

Transition to Carnivore: Skeptical yet desperate, Alexandra decided to give the carnivore diet a try after reading its potential benefits.

Outcome: Within months, her energy levels surged. Now, she's an active hiker, a passionate dancer, and most importantly, free from the chains of constant fatigue.

Liam's Weight Loss Journey

Background: Liam's struggle with obesity began in childhood. By his late 20s, he weighed over 300 lbs and was diagnosed with type 2 diabetes.

Transition to Carnivore: Inspired by success stories online, Liam adopted the carnivore diet, focusing mainly on lean meats.

Outcome: Over the span of two years, Liam shed 130 lbs, reversed his diabetes, and gained a newfound confidence.

Priya's Combat Against Autoimmune Disorders

Background: Priya was diagnosed with multiple autoimmune disorders in her early 30s. Flare-ups, pain, and medication became a regular part of her life.

Transition to Carnivore: After researching dietary interventions, Priya stumbled upon the carnivore diet. With a glimmer of hope, she transitioned.

Outcome: Today, Priya's flare-ups are rare, her medication has drastically reduced, and she believes her diet plays a significant role in her improved health.

Carlos' Mental Health Breakthrough

Background: Carlos always felt under the cloud of depression and anxiety. Despite therapy and medication, the fog never fully lifted.

Transition to Carnivore: A friend's recommendation led Carlos to the carnivore diet. Initially skeptical, he was surprised by the results.

Outcome: Not only does Carlos feel more energetic, but he also mentions a newfound mental clarity and reduced bouts of anxiety.

These are just snapshots of countless individuals who've reaped profound changes by embracing the carnivore lifestyle. While results vary, and it's crucial to approach any diet with research and consultation, these stories showcase the potential positive impacts of an all-meat diet.

Challenges Faced and How They Were Overcome

Adopting a carnivore diet, like any significant lifestyle shift, comes with its own set of challenges. Here are some real-life accounts of the obstacles individuals encountered on this journey and the innovative ways they tackled them:

Maria's Social Dining Dilemma

Challenge: Maria loved dining out with friends. Transitioning to a carnivore diet made her feel isolated during social gatherings, with limited food choices that matched her new lifestyle.

Solution: Maria started researching and shortlisting carnivore-friendly restaurants. She also initiated a monthly 'meat-up' – a social gathering where everyone either followed the carnivore diet or was carnivore-curious. It became a hit!

Ahmed's Financial Constraints

Challenge: Ahmed, a college student, found the carnivore diet appealing but struggled with the costs associated with sourcing quality meats.

Solution: Ahmed delved into bulk-buying, freezing meat, and also became a frequent visitor to local farmers' markets during discount hours. He learned the art of using cheaper cuts and organs, which are nutrient-dense yet budget-friendly.

Sasha's Initial Fatigue

Challenge: During her first few weeks on the carnivore diet, Sasha felt unusually tired and considered quitting.

Solution: Sasha discovered the 'adaptation phase,' where initial fatigue or 'keto flu' is common. She increased her intake of electrolytes and ensured she consumed enough fats. Gradually, her energy levels stabilized.

Jin's Boredom with Food Choices

Challenge: Jin, a culinary enthusiast, initially felt the carnivore diet was monotonous.

Solution: Jin began experimenting with different meat-based recipes, incorporating various cooking techniques, and exploring less common meats and organ products. His culinary passion reignited, making his meals both nutritious and exciting.

Elena's Criticism from Friends and Family

Challenge: Elena's decision to adopt the carnivore diet was met with skepticism and criticism from loved ones, causing her to second-guess her choice.

Solution: Elena equipped herself with knowledge. She read extensively on the topic, joined online carnivore communities, and even attended seminars. Being well-informed, she was better at addressing concerns and even inspired a few friends to give it a try.

Lucas' Travel Constraints

Challenge: Being a frequent traveler, Lucas found it challenging to maintain his carnivore regimen on the road.

Solution: Lucas started packing jerky, canned fish, and other portable meat items. He also researched his destinations in advance for local butcher shops and carnivore-friendly eateries. His trips became an opportunity to explore new meat-based dishes from different cultures.

These narratives underscore a crucial point: while challenges are inevitable in any journey, they are surmountable with determination, creativity, and a dash of resourcefulness.

Before-and-After Comparisons

Change is the only constant, they say. And when individuals make a substantial shift in their diet, the results can often be stark and telling. Here are some striking before-and-after accounts of those who embraced the carnivore lifestyle:

Anna's Weight Journey

Before: At 220 lbs, Anna struggled with her self-image, frequent joint pains, and fatigue.

After: Six months into the carnivore diet, Anna dropped to 170 lbs. Not only did her confidence surge, but her joint pains vanished, and her energy levels peaked.

Bryan's Battle with Digestive Issues

Before: Bryan often grappled with bloating, gas, and unpredictable bowel movements, making him apprehensive about dining out.

After: A consistent carnivore diet for four months cleared Bryan's digestive woes. Dining out became a joy as he no longer had to worry about surprise flare-ups.

Clara's Skin Transformation

Before: Acne outbreaks and inconsistent skin tone made Clara invest heavily in cosmetics and skin treatments, often to little avail.

After: Three months into her new diet, Clara's skin began to clear up. The redness reduced, and acne became a rare occurrence. She now confidently steps out with minimal makeup.

Derrick's Mental Clarity

Before: Derrick frequently battled brain fog, making it challenging to focus on tasks and often resulting in unproductive days.

After: Embracing the carnivore diet, Derrick found a renewed sense of clarity. Tasks that earlier seemed daunting were now tackled with ease and efficiency.

Eve's Blood Sugar Control

Before: As a Type 2 diabetic, Eve's fluctuating blood sugar levels were a constant concern, despite medication.

After: Post transition to the carnivore diet, not only did Eve's blood sugar levels stabilize, but she was also able to reduce her medication dosage with her doctor's approval.

Franco's Gym Performance

Before: Franco, an avid gym-goer, often felt his performance plateaued. Muscle gain was slow, and recovery took longer.

After: On the carnivore diet, Franco experienced improved muscle definition, increased strength, and reduced post-workout recovery times.

These compelling transformations highlight the multifaceted benefits that the carnivore diet can offer, touching various aspects of physical and mental well-being.

Chapter 9

The Role of Exercise with the Carnivore Diet

Exercise and diet – two pillars that often walk hand in hand when we talk about achieving optimal health. Just as a car runs best with quality fuel, our bodies, too, require the right nutrition to perform at their peak. The carnivore diet, rich in proteins and fats, has been hailed by many for its myriad benefits. But where does exercise fit into this dietary equation? Can a meat-centric diet complement your fitness routine? Or is there more to the story that we need to explore?

In this chapter, we will dive deep into the synergy between the carnivore diet and physical activity. Whether you're an athlete aiming for peak performance or someone just looking to stay active and healthy, understanding how this diet interacts with your workouts can be the key to unlocking new milestones.

Join us as we unravel the dynamics of muscle building, endurance, recovery, and more, all under the lens of the carnivore diet.

Adapting Workout Routines

When embarking on a dietary shift like the carnivore diet, it's not just your meals that might need some tweaking. Your workout routine, too, may benefit from some adjustments to align better with your new nutritional intake. The carnivore diet, primarily centered on animal products, is protein-rich and can offer a unique fuel source for your workouts.

Understanding Energy Sources

The carnivore diet is predominantly low in carbohydrates. Unlike traditional diets where carbs are the primary energy source, here, your body might turn to fats and proteins. This means during workouts, especially high-intensity ones, you might experience an initial drop in stamina as your body adjusts to using fats as a primary energy source.

Embracing Strength Training

Given the protein-rich nature of the carnivore diet, it's an excellent opportunity to focus on muscle building and strength training. Consuming ample protein can aid in muscle recovery and growth. Consider incorporating more weightlifting sessions, resistance bands, and bodyweight exercises into your regimen.

Modifying Cardio Sessions

While cardio remains an essential component of overall fitness, those on the carnivore diet might notice a shift in their endurance levels, especially in the beginning. It might be worth adjusting the intensity or duration of your cardio sessions as your body gets used to its new fuel source.

Prioritizing Recovery:

With an abundant supply of amino acids from the meat, your body is well-equipped to repair and rebuild muscles post-workout. Ensure you're giving your body enough rest between workouts, and consider incorporating stretching or yoga to aid in recovery.

Listening to Your Body

Every individual's response to the carnivore diet can vary. While some might feel an energy surge, others might take time to adjust. It's crucial to listen to your body's signals. If you feel fatigued or notice a drop in performance, consider consulting with a fitness expert or nutritionist familiar with the carnivore diet.

Experiment and Adjust

The beauty of fitness routines lies in their adaptability. As you progress on the carnivore diet, continually assess and tweak your workout routines. Experimenting will help you find the sweet spot that complements your dietary choices.

Strength Training vs. Cardio Considerations on the Carnivore Diet

Navigating the fitness world while on the carnivore diet requires understanding how the diet interacts with different workout modalities. Given the diet's heavy emphasis on protein and fat with little to no carbohydrates, it can influence the way our body responds to strength training and cardio. Let's delve deeper into how one might approach these two essential pillars of fitness while on the carnivore diet.

Strength Training on a Carnivore Diet

Protein as an Ally: The carnivore diet is inherently rich in proteins. This makes it advantageous for muscle repair, recovery, and growth. After a strength training session, the proteins consumed can help in the quicker recovery of torn muscle fibers.

Fat for Fuel: In the absence of carbohydrates, the body turns to fats as a primary energy source. This can be beneficial for longer, lower-intensity strength training sessions where stored fat can be utilized effectively.

Enhanced Muscle Mass: With an adequate supply of essential amino acids from meat consumption, individuals on the carnivore diet might experience a more pronounced muscle mass gain over time, provided they're engaging in consistent resistance training.

Cardio on a Carnivore Diet

Initial Energy Dip: With carbs typically acting as the primary energy source during high-intensity cardio, those on the carnivore diet might initially experience reduced stamina. Over time, however, the body adapts to utilizing fat more efficiently, which can sustain longer, moderate-intensity cardio sessions.

Fat Adaptation: As the body becomes more accustomed to burning fats for energy—a state often referred to as being "fat-adapted"—one might find improved endurance for activities like long-distance running, cycling, or swimming.

Intensity Considerations: High-intensity interval training (HIIT) relies heavily on carbohydrate stores. While it's possible to engage in HIIT on the carnivore diet, some might find it beneficial to adjust the intensity or duration of such workouts, especially in the initial transition phase.

Balancing Both

Fueling Workouts: It's essential to ensure that you're consuming enough calories, particularly on workout days. This can mean eating larger meat portions or incorporating fattier cuts to sustain both strength and cardio workouts.

Recovery: Regardless of the workout type, recovery remains crucial. The carnivore diet can aid this due to its anti-inflammatory potential and rich protein content. However, ensure you're getting ample rest and staying hydrated.

Personalization is Key
Every individual's experience on the carnivore diet will differ. Some might find they thrive more on strength training, while others might excel in their cardio pursuits. The key is to experiment, listen to your body, and adjust accordingly.

In conclusion, while the carnivore diet poses certain considerations for strength training and cardio, with informed choices and listening to one's body, it's entirely possible to find a balance that promotes overall health and fitness.

Recovery and Muscle Growth on a Meat-Only Diet

When it comes to athletic performance, recovery, and muscle growth, diet plays a pivotal role. The carnivore or meat-only diet offers a unique nutritional profile that can significantly influence these factors. Let's delve deep into understanding how a meat-centric diet can impact recovery and muscle development.

Amino Acids Galore

Protein Powerhouse: Meat is a complete protein source, meaning it provides all the essential amino acids the body needs. Amino acids are the building blocks of proteins, crucial for repairing muscle tissue and promoting muscle growth.

Direct Benefit: After intense workouts, especially strength training, our muscles undergo wear and tear. The abundant protein supply from a meat-only diet provides ample amino acids to expedite the repair process, aiding faster recovery and promoting muscle synthesis.

Anti-inflammatory Potential

Omega-3 Fatty Acids: Certain meats, especially fatty fish like salmon, are rich in omega-3 fatty acids, known for their anti-inflammatory properties. Reduced inflammation can lead to quicker recovery post-workout.

Less Plant Antinutrients: Advocates of the carnivore diet argue that by eliminating plant-based foods, you reduce the intake of certain compounds that can cause inflammation in some people, potentially enhancing recovery.

Fat as Fuel

Metabolic Shift: On a meat-only diet, the body shifts to using fat as a primary energy source. This metabolic adaptation can provide sustained energy for workouts, reducing muscle fatigue, and potentially leading to more effective training sessions.

Ketosis and Muscle Preservation: If carbohydrate intake is minimal, the body might enter a state of ketosis, where it burns fat for energy. There's evidence suggesting that being in ketosis can have muscle-sparing effects, meaning the body is less likely to break down muscle tissue for energy.

Nutrient Density

Rich in Minerals: Meat is dense in essential minerals like zinc, iron, and magnesium, which play roles in muscle function, protein synthesis, and recovery.

Vitamins for Recovery: Meat provides essential vitamins, especially B-vitamins, which assist in energy production and the formation of red blood cells, enhancing oxygen delivery to muscles.

Considerations and Recommendations

Stay Hydrated: A meat-only diet can be diuretic, meaning it might cause increased urine production. Staying hydrated is crucial for muscle function and recovery.

Diverse Meat Selection: To maximize benefits, ensure a variety of meats are consumed. While muscle meat (like steaks) is valuable, don't neglect organ meats, which are nutrient powerhouses.

Monitor and Adjust: As with any diet, individual responses will vary. It's essential to monitor how your body reacts, especially concerning recovery times and muscle growth. Adjust meat types, quantities, and workout regimens accordingly.

In conclusion, a meat-only diet offers several attributes conducive to muscle recovery and growth. The high protein content, anti-inflammatory potential, and nutrient density of meat can support athletes and fitness enthusiasts in their training goals. However, as always, it's essential to approach it informed and in tune with one's body.

Chapter 10

Carnivore Diet in Special Situations

Every individual is a unique blend of genetics, environment, and personal history, and thus, their nutritional needs and responses to diets can vary. While the carnivore diet's fundamental principle remains consistent—consuming primarily, if not exclusively, animal products—special situations require additional considerations. From pregnancy and lactation to endurance sports or handling specific medical conditions, it's vital to understand how the carnivore diet might interact, support, or need adaptations. This chapter sheds light on navigating the carnivore diet during these particular scenarios, ensuring safety, health, and optimal benefits. It's an exploration into the flexible facets of an otherwise seemingly strict dietary approach.

Pregnancy and Breastfeeding on the Carnivore Diet

Pregnancy and breastfeeding are two of the most transformative periods in a woman's life. The body's requirements shift, placing a greater emphasis on specific nutrients to support the growth of the baby and the health of the mother. When considering the carnivore diet during these stages, a few key considerations come into play.

Nutritional Needs
During pregnancy, the demand for certain nutrients, such as iron, folic acid, and calcium, increases. A carnivore diet, rich in meats, can provide ample iron. Liver, a highly recommended organ meat on this diet, is a potent source of folate, although it's different from the folic acid found in most prenatal vitamins. Calcium can be sourced from small, edible bones, like those in sardines or from bone broth.

Essential Fatty Acids
DHA, a type of omega-3 fatty acid, plays a crucial role in the baby's brain development. While fish is the most commonly known source, those on a strict carnivore diet can also obtain DHA from grass-fed meats and organ meats like liver.

Protein Intake

Protein is a cornerstone of the carnivore diet, and it's vital during pregnancy for cell growth. However, moderation is key. Excessive protein can put a strain on the kidneys, so balance and listening to the body's cues are essential.

Hydration and Electrolytes

Pregnant women on a carnivore diet should be especially mindful of their hydration levels. As the diet is naturally diuretic, consuming enough water and ensuring a balance of electrolytes is crucial.

Breastfeeding Considerations

While the carnivore diet can be nutrient-dense, breast milk composition can vary based on maternal diet. Mothers should monitor their baby's reactions (like fussiness or rashes) that could indicate a sensitivity or intolerance to something in the milk.

Listening to Your Body

Every woman's experience with pregnancy and breastfeeding is unique. Some might find they crave certain plant foods during this time. Honoring those cravings, especially if they're for nutrient-dense plant foods, can be considered.

Consultation

Before making any drastic dietary changes during pregnancy or breastfeeding, it's imperative to consult with a healthcare professional. They can provide guidance tailored to individual needs and monitor both maternal and fetal health.

In conclusion, while the carnivore diet can be maintained during pregnancy and breastfeeding, careful planning and attention to the body's signals are crucial. It's a period where the mother's and baby's health should be the top priority, and flexibility in dietary choices can be beneficial.

Athletes and High-Performance Individuals on the Carnivore Diet

The world of sports and high-performance activities demands optimal nutrition to fuel rigorous training, support recovery, and enhance overall performance. Athletes, from marathon runners to weightlifters, have specific dietary needs. The carnivore diet's emphasis on animal-based nutrition presents both potential advantages and challenges for these individuals.

Protein for Muscle Growth and Repair

For athletes, protein is essential. It aids in muscle repair, growth, and overall maintenance. The carnivore diet is inherently high in protein, offering a direct source from meats which could benefit muscle synthesis and recovery.

Fat as Fuel

On a typical diet, carbohydrates serve as the primary energy source. However, a carnivore diet shifts this paradigm, making fat the primary energy source. This could be advantageous for endurance athletes, as fats provide a more sustained energy release compared to quick-burning carbohydrates.

Electrolyte Balance

The importance of electrolytes, such as sodium, potassium, and magnesium, can't be overstated for athletes. The carnivore diet can be naturally low in some of these, so attention to adequate intake, possibly from bone broths or supplements, is crucial, especially for those engaging in prolonged or intense physical activity.

Adaptation Period

Switching to a carnivore diet means transitioning to fat as the primary energy source. This change can initially lead to decreased performance, often termed as the "low-carb flu." Athletes should be prepared for this transition phase, which can last a few days to several weeks.

Considerations for Explosive Activities

While endurance athletes might benefit from the sustained energy from fats, those in sports requiring short, explosive bursts (like sprinting or weightlifting) might miss the quick energy from carbohydrates. Some athletes incorporate targeted carb intake, aligning with their training to reap the benefits of both worlds.

Recovery and Inflammation

Some athletes on the carnivore diet report faster recovery times and reduced inflammation. While anecdotal, this could be due to the elimination of potential inflammatory plant compounds from the diet.

Nutrient Timing

In traditional sports nutrition, there's a significant emphasis on nutrient timing, especially around workouts. On the carnivore diet, this might be less pronounced, but athletes should still pay attention to their protein intake post-workout for optimal recovery.

Listening to the Body

Athletes, more than anyone, are tuned into their bodies. It's essential to monitor performance, recovery, and overall well-being when on the carnivore diet, adjusting as necessary.

Individual Variation

What works for one athlete might not work for another. The carnivore diet could be a game-changer for some, while others might find they perform better with some plant-based foods included.

In conclusion, while the carnivore diet presents a radical shift from traditional sports nutrition, it offers potential benefits for athletes and high-performance individuals. However, careful planning, listening to the body, and possibly making hybrid dietary choices can ensure they meet their performance and health goals.

Managing Social Situations and Dining Out on the Carnivore Diet

Choosing a specialized diet often brings its own set of challenges, especially when faced with social situations and dining out. The carnivore diet, with its focus solely on animal-based foods, is no exception. However, with a bit of planning, understanding, and flexibility, navigating these situations can become much more manageable.

Communication is Key

If you're attending a gathering or party, it's helpful to let the host know about your dietary preferences ahead of time. This not only prevents potential awkward situations but might also ensure there's something you can eat.

BYOM (Bring Your Own Meat)

In casual gatherings or BBQs, consider bringing your own meat. This way, you can be sure of what you're eating, and it often becomes a conversation starter, allowing you to share about your dietary choices.

Explore the Menu in Advance

Most restaurants post their menus online. Before heading out, check to see if there are suitable carnivore options. Steakhouses, seafood places, and grill restaurants are often the best bets.

Customization

Don't be afraid to ask for modifications to menu items. For instance, a burger can be ordered without the bun and veggies, or a salad can be turned into a meat-based dish.

Avoiding Awkwardness

There will always be individuals who question or even criticize dietary choices. Prepare a brief and non-confrontational response about why you've chosen the carnivore diet. Being prepared can defuse potential tension.

Always Have a Snack

Carrying a small snack, like beef jerky or a can of tuna, can be a lifesaver if you find yourself in situations where there's nothing carnivore-friendly on the menu.

Flexibility in Limited Scenarios

If you're in a situation where sticking strictly to the carnivore diet is challenging, decide in advance how flexible you're willing to be. For some, having a non-carnivore item once in a while is okay, especially if it helps manage social situations smoothly.

Drinks and Beverages

While water is the go-to, other drinks might contain hidden sugars or plant-based ingredients. If you're consuming alcohol, opt for clear spirits and avoid mixers that might have sugars or juices.

Be Prepared for Curiosity

The carnivore diet is still relatively new to many, and people are bound to be curious. Use this as an opportunity to educate and share, but also be understanding that it might seem radical to some.

Respect Others' Choices

Just as you'd like others to respect your dietary choices, be sure to offer the same courtesy to others. Everyone has their reasons for eating the way they do.

In summary, while the carnivore diet can introduce some challenges in social and dining-out scenarios, they're not insurmountable. With a mix of planning, communication, and flexibility, you can stick to your dietary choices and still enjoy a rich social life.

Chapter 11

Addressing Common Misconceptions

In the world of nutrition and diet, misconceptions are as plentiful as the diverse array of eating habits. This is particularly true for diets that veer off the traditional path, such as the carnivore diet. But as with all subjects, understanding is essential to dispelling myths and shedding light on the truth.

The carnivore diet, emphasizing animal-based foods while excluding most, if not all, plant-based foods, naturally raises eyebrows and questions. Some wonder about its health implications, while others question its sustainability. Many of these concerns stem from long-held beliefs about nutrition and health.

In this chapter, we'll dive deep into some of the most common misconceptions surrounding the carnivore diet. We aim to provide clarity, armed with facts, research, and practical experiences, to help both enthusiasts and skeptics alike navigate the sea of information and opinions about this unique dietary approach. By addressing these misconceptions head-on, we hope to pave the way for a more informed, open dialogue about the carnivore diet's role in modern nutrition.

Challenging Anti-Meat Propaganda

Historical Perspective

For decades, meat, especially red meat, has often been portrayed negatively in various media channels, linking it to health issues ranging from heart disease to cancer. This portrayal, in many cases, can be traced back to dietary guidelines and influential studies from the 20th century. One such instance was the Seven Countries Study led by Ancel Keys in the 1950s, which suggested a correlation between saturated fat intake and heart disease. Though the methodology and conclusions of this study have since been challenged, its influence has persisted.

The Nuances of Nutritional Science

It's crucial to understand that nutrition is a complex field, and boiling it down to "good" or "bad" food categories is an oversimplification. Many anti-meat studies often rely on observational data, which can identify correlations but not causations. For instance, while some studies have found a correlation between meat consumption and certain diseases, they often don't account for other lifestyle factors such as smoking, lack of exercise, or overall dietary patterns.

Quality and Processing Matters

Another point of contention in anti-meat propaganda is the blanket categorization of all meat as being the same. Processed meats, like sausages and bacon, which often contain additives, are different from whole, unprocessed cuts of meat. Many studies that point to the detrimental effects of meat consumption do not distinguish between these types, leading to generalized conclusions.

Environmental Concerns and Ethical Farming

The environmental impact of meat production is another angle from which meat consumption has been criticized. While there's no denying that certain methods of meat production, especially in factory farms, can be environmentally taxing, it's worth noting that sustainable farming practices present a viable solution. Grass-fed and pasture-raised animals, for instance, can play a role in ecosystem balance, promoting soil health and carbon sequestration.

Moreover, ethical considerations about animal welfare have spurred on the anti-meat narrative. While these concerns are valid, they address the methods of production rather than the consumption of meat per se. Ethical farming practices, which prioritize animal welfare, offer a middle-ground solution.

Balanced Perspective: Benefits of Meat

In challenging the anti-meat narrative, it's also worth highlighting the undeniable nutritional benefits of meat. Rich in essential nutrients like iron, vitamin B12, and high-quality proteins, meat can be a valuable part of a balanced diet. For certain populations, especially those with specific dietary restrictions or health conditions, meat can provide vital nutrients that might be challenging to obtain elsewhere.

Conclusion

While it's essential to approach all dietary decisions with a critical mind, it's equally crucial to differentiate between informed critiques and generalized propaganda. By delving deep into the research, understanding the nuances, and recognizing the value of quality and ethical considerations, one can make more informed choices about meat consumption and its place in a balanced diet.

Clarifying Myths About Cholesterol, Saturated Fats, and Heart Disease

Historical Background

For many decades, cholesterol and saturated fats have been demonized, largely due to their alleged association with heart disease. This perspective mainly stemmed from influential studies like the Seven Countries Study, which observed correlations between saturated fat intake and heart disease rates. As a result, dietary guidelines worldwide began recommending reduced intake of saturated fats.

Cholesterol: The Basics

Dietary vs. Serum Cholesterol: One common misconception is that eating cholesterol-rich foods directly raises blood cholesterol levels. However, dietary cholesterol (found in food) has a minimal effect on serum cholesterol (in the bloodstream). The liver produces most of the body's cholesterol, and when dietary intake increases, liver production typically decreases.

HDL vs. LDL Cholesterol: Not all cholesterol is the same. HDL (high-density lipoprotein) is often termed "good" cholesterol, as it can remove cholesterol from blood vessels. LDL (low-density lipoprotein), often termed "bad" cholesterol, can lead to plaque build-up in arteries. However, there's more nuance; particle size matters, with small, dense LDL particles being more atherogenic than larger ones.

Saturated Fats and Heart Disease: The Debate

Inconsistent Evidence: Contrary to popular belief, the link between saturated fats and heart disease isn't unanimous. Numerous recent meta-analyses have found no significant association between saturated fat intake and heart disease risk.

Context Matters: Not all saturated fats are the same, and their sources vary (dairy, meat, tropical oils). Their effects can differ based on the overall dietary context. For instance, while trans fats (a type of unsaturated fat) are harmful, saturated fats from whole foods like dairy might even have protective effects.

Reevaluating the "Fat Hypothesis"

Carbohydrates and Sugar: With the demonization of fats, many turned to high-carb, low-fat diets. There's increasing evidence that excessive refined carb and sugar intake can be more detrimental to heart health, leading to conditions like insulin resistance, obesity, and type 2 diabetes, which are significant heart disease risk factors.

Dietary Patterns Over Single Nutrients: Focusing solely on single nutrients, like saturated fats, is an oversimplification. Dietary patterns, such as the Mediterranean diet, which may include saturated fats but also emphasizes fruits, vegetables, and whole grains, have been shown to be beneficial for heart health.

Individual Variation

Genetic Factors: Genetic factors can influence how different individuals metabolize and respond to dietary fats. Some people might be "hyper-responders" to dietary cholesterol, while others are not.

The Role of Inflammation: Chronic inflammation is now recognized as a significant factor in heart disease. Rather than saturated fat per se, diets high in processed foods, trans fats, and sugars might drive inflammation, contributing to heart disease risk.

Conclusion
The narrative surrounding cholesterol, saturated fats, and heart disease is more complex than previously thought. While it's essential to be cautious about excessive saturated fat intake, especially from processed sources, it's equally critical to view these nutrients within the broader context of overall diet, lifestyle, and individual variation.

Chapter 12

Frequently Asked Questions (FAQs)

As we delve deeper into the world of the carnivore diet, it's only natural that questions arise. Whether you're just embarking on this journey or have been on the path for some time, uncertainties and curiosities are part and parcel of adopting any new lifestyle. This chapter is dedicated to addressing some of the most common and pressing queries about the carnivore diet. From its effects on specific health conditions to day-to-day practicalities, we've compiled and answered a series of frequently asked questions to shed light on areas you might be pondering. Let's set the record straight and dive into the answers you've been seeking!

Digestive Changes: Lack of Fiber, Bowel Movements, etc.

One of the most frequently broached subjects when discussing the carnivore diet revolves around digestion. Considering that the diet is devoid of plant-based sources, it prompts questions about the impact on our digestive system, notably due to the absence of fiber. Let's explore these concerns in detail.

The Role of Fiber in Traditional Diets

In a standard diet, fiber is championed for its role in promoting regular bowel movements and supporting gut health. It's known to add bulk to stools, aiding in their passage through the digestive system.

The Carnivore Diet and Fiber

When you shift to a carnivore diet, the intake of dietary fiber drops to nearly zero. However, many adherents of the diet claim that, contrary to popular belief, they still experience regular and unproblematic bowel movements. This challenges the common notion that fiber is an essential component for digestive regularity.

Bowel Movement Changes

Initially, as with any drastic dietary change, individuals may experience changes in their bowel habits. This can range from constipation to loose stools. However, over time, many report a stabilization where they might go less frequently but without discomfort or issues.

Stool Volume and Composition

Given that meat is more densely nutritious and less bulky than plant matter, the volume of stool generally decreases on a carnivore diet. The body absorbs a higher proportion of animal-based foods, leaving behind less waste.

Gut Flora Adaptations

The human gut is a dynamic environment, housing a myriad of bacteria that play essential roles in our overall health. The shift to a meat-only diet will inevitably change the composition of this gut microbiome. Some studies suggest that while there's a shift in the bacterial populations, it doesn't necessarily equate to an unhealthy gut environment. The optimal gut flora for a carnivore diet may simply be different from that of a mixed or plant-based diet.

Potential Benefits and Concerns

Some carnivore diet followers report improved symptoms of bloating, gas, and other digestive discomforts that they experienced on their previous diets. On the flip side, if an individual doesn't transition properly or doesn't consume a balanced variety of animal foods, they might face challenges like constipation. Hydration and the intake of fats play crucial roles in mitigating such issues.

Conclusion

Digestive changes are a natural part of adapting to the carnivore diet. While the absence of fiber might seem concerning initially, many individuals find that their bodies adjust over time, maintaining digestive health and regularity. As with any dietary modification, it's essential to monitor one's body's responses and seek expert advice if any issues persist.

Dealing with Cravings for Plant-Based Foods

Transitioning to a carnivore diet means leaving behind the flavors, textures, and comfort of plant-based foods that many have enjoyed for most of their lives. This can lead to powerful cravings, especially during the initial phase. Let's explore why these cravings occur and how to navigate them.

Why Cravings Occur

Memory and Comfort: Foods, especially our favorites, are not just about nourishment. They hold memories, rituals, and emotions. A specific dish might remind us of family gatherings or celebrations.

Sugar and Carbs: Many plant-based foods, especially processed ones, contain sugars and carbs that can lead to a sort of addiction. When deprived of them, our body can crave these quick energy sources.

Gut Bacteria: The gut microbiome, which thrives on various nutrients from plant-based foods, can influence our cravings. As the balance of bacteria shifts, so can our desires for certain foods.

Strategies to Overcome Cravings

Stay Satiated: Ensure you're eating enough on the carnivore diet. A full belly can significantly reduce the temptation of cravings.

Healthy Fat Intake: Incorporating a good amount of healthy animal fats can help in feeling satisfied and provide a steady energy source, reducing the need for quick energy from sugars and carbs.

Distraction: Sometimes, cravings are more about boredom or emotional needs rather than hunger. Engage in an activity, take a walk, or practice deep breathing.

Hydration: Drinking enough water can sometimes help in curbing cravings. Occasionally, our bodies confuse thirst with hunger.

Spices and Seasonings: While purists might stick to salt, others find that using various seasonings (without additives) can help satiate the palate's need for diverse flavors.

Gradual Transition: Instead of diving straight into a strict carnivore diet, some people find it beneficial to transition slowly, phasing out plant-based foods gradually.

Understanding the Difference Between Cravings and Nutritional Needs

Sometimes, a craving might be the body's way of signaling a nutritional need. It's essential to differentiate between wanting a food for emotional comfort and requiring a nutrient that might be missing in the diet. For instance, craving chocolate might indicate a magnesium deficiency.

Mental and Emotional Approaches

Mindful Eating: Pay attention to each bite. Savor the flavors of the meat and connect with the act of eating. This can reduce feelings of deprivation.

Positive Affirmations: Reminding oneself about the health goals and benefits of the carnivore diet can help in staying on track.

Community Support: Engaging with online communities or support groups following the carnivore diet can provide encouragement, tips, and a sense of belonging.

Conclusion

Cravings are a natural part of transitioning to a new way of eating. However, with understanding, strategy, and support, they can be managed and even reduced over time. Embracing the journey and being kind to oneself during moments of temptation is key.

Traveling and Maintaining the Carnivore Lifestyle

Traveling can often disrupt our usual routines, from sleep patterns to workout regimens, and, of course, our diet. When you're committed to the carnivore lifestyle, hopping from one city to another or jetting off to a foreign country can present challenges in staying true to this dietary choice. But with some forethought and flexibility, maintaining the carnivore diet while traveling can be entirely achievable.

Preparation is Key

Research Your Destination: Before setting off, spend some time investigating the local cuisine. Many cultures have meat-centric dishes that can easily fit into a carnivore diet. Know these dishes and have a list ready.

Pack Snacks: Carry carnivore-friendly snacks such as jerky, canned fish, or boiled eggs. They can be lifesavers during long transit times or in places where carnivore options aren't readily available.

Hotel Choices: If possible, book accommodations with kitchen facilities. This gives you the flexibility to cook your own meals, ensuring they align with your dietary preferences.

Eating Out

Steakhouses and Grill Restaurants: These are your best friends. Most cities will have a steakhouse or a grill-centric restaurant that can cater to your needs.

Customize Your Order: Don't be shy about asking for modifications. For instance, at a burger joint, you can request a bunless burger. Similarly, in many restaurants, you can swap out plant-based sides for an extra serving of meat or animal-based sides.

Language Barriers: If you're in a country where you don't speak the language, have a translation app or a small card that explains your dietary choices. This can help restaurant staff cater to your needs.

Be Flexible and Kind to Yourself

Perfect vs. Good Enough: While you might strive for 100% adherence to the carnivore diet at home, it's essential to accept that while traveling, 80% or 90% might sometimes have to do. The experience of travel is also about exploring new cultures, including their culinary traditions.

Intermittent Fasting: If you find yourself in a situation where there are no suitable food options, consider intermittent fasting until you find your next carnivore-friendly meal.

Embrace Local Delicacies

Many regions have unique animal-based delicacies. From the seafood delights of coastal areas to specific regional cured meats or cheeses, there's often something new and exciting for the carnivorous traveler to try.

Stay Hydrated

Especially during long flights or train journeys, it's easy to get dehydrated. Carry a reusable water bottle and keep drinking. This not only keeps you hydrated but can also help curb hunger pangs.

Supplements and Medications

If you take specific supplements as part of your carnivore lifestyle, ensure you pack enough for your trip's duration. Also, always check the travel regulations regarding carrying supplements and medicines.

Conclusion

While maintaining a strict dietary regimen like the carnivore diet can seem daunting on the road, it's more than possible with a bit of preparation and flexibility. Embrace the journey, enjoy the local carnivore-friendly offerings, and remember why you chose this lifestyle in the first place.

Chapter 13

Conclusion

The Future of the Carnivore Movement

The carnivore diet, which emphasizes consuming primarily animal-based foods and avoiding plant-based ones, has seen a notable surge in recent years. As with any dietary movement, there's a mixture of skepticism, enthusiasm, and curiosity surrounding it. However, considering the ongoing global shifts in nutrition, health, and environmental consciousness, what might the future hold for the carnivore movement?

Increased Scientific Research

Demand for Evidence: The modern world increasingly relies on evidence-based approaches to health and wellness. As more people experiment with the carnivore diet, there will likely be a surge in scientific research to understand its long-term benefits and drawbacks.

Clarifying Myths: More rigorous studies can help dispel myths and misinformation around diets high in meat consumption, especially concerning cholesterol, heart diseases, and overall longevity.

Environmental Debates

Sustainability Issues: Critics often point out the environmental concerns related to large-scale meat production, from deforestation to greenhouse gas emissions. As the carnivore movement grows, these debates will intensify.

Regenerative Agriculture: On the flip side, advocates highlight the potential benefits of regenerative farming practices that can be more sustainable and environmentally friendly. The future might see a shift toward such practices if demand for meat continues to rise.

Innovations in Meat Production

Lab-grown Meat: With advancements in technology, lab-grown or cultured meats could become a significant part of our dietary landscape. If accepted by the carnivore community, this could be a game-changer in addressing both ethical and environmental concerns.

Alternative Animal Products: The market may see an increase in products like insect proteins or other less conventional animal-based foods, expanding the options for those on a carnivore diet.

Expansion of the Global Community

Online Platforms: The internet has played a pivotal role in the growth of the carnivore movement, allowing like-minded individuals to share experiences, recipes, and advice. We can expect this global community to flourish, with more forums, blogs, podcasts, and YouTube channels dedicated to the lifestyle.

Celebrity Endorsements: As more public figures and athletes attribute their health or performance improvements to the carnivore diet, this could boost its popularity further.

Adaptations and Variations

Hybrid Approaches: As people personalize the diet to their needs, we might see more variations that include limited plant foods or specific supplementation, much like the evolution of other dietary approaches.

Cultural Incorporation: Different cultures may adapt the carnivore diet according to their traditional foods and culinary practices, leading to diverse global interpretations of the diet.

While predicting the exact trajectory of any movement can be challenging, the carnivore diet's future will likely be shaped by scientific research, environmental considerations, technological innovations, and cultural factors.

Continued Research and Evolving Perspectives

The world of nutrition is ever-evolving, and our understanding of diets and their impacts on health is no exception. The carnivore diet, a relatively new player in the nutrition arena, is part of this dynamic landscape. As more individuals adopt and advocate for this way of eating, there's an increased demand for rigorous scientific research to validate or challenge its claims.

Areas of Investigation

Long-Term Health Impacts: While short-term studies and anecdotal evidence suggest various benefits of the carnivore diet, long-term studies are essential. These will address concerns related to heart health, bone density, and potential nutrient deficiencies.

Mental Health and Cognitive Function: Emerging evidence suggests that diet plays a pivotal role in mental well-being and cognitive performance. Understanding how a meat-centric diet influences brain health and function will be a valuable avenue of exploration.

Gut Health: Traditional thought emphasizes the role of dietary fiber in gut health. Research on how an all-meat diet, devoid of traditional fiber sources, impacts the microbiome and overall digestive health will provide clearer insights.

Expanding the Participant Pool

Diverse Demographics: Initial studies often involve specific demographics. To have a holistic understanding, research should include diverse age groups, ethnicities, and medical histories.

Special Populations: Understanding the diet's impact on athletes, pregnant or breastfeeding women, and those with specific medical conditions will further solidify its applicability.

Evolving Nutritional Perspectives

Challenging Established Norms: Traditional dietary guidelines emphasize balanced meals from various food groups. The carnivore diet, emphasizing primarily animal products, challenges these norms, prompting a re-evaluation of what "balanced" truly means.

Interdisciplinary Approaches: Collaboration between nutritionists, anthropologists, environmental scientists, and other experts can offer a 360-degree perspective on the diet's sustainability, health impacts, and socio-cultural implications.

Integration with Modern Technology

Data Tracking: With wearable tech and apps that monitor various health metrics, it's easier than ever for individuals to track their progress and health changes. This real-time data can be invaluable for researchers.

Genetics and Personalization: As we advance in understanding genetics, research might delve into how one's genes can influence their response to the carnivore diet.

Conclusion

The future of the carnivore diet isn't just in the anecdotes of its proponents but also in the labs, clinics, and research centers where its effects are studied objectively. As with all dietary practices, the carnivore diet will likely see adaptations and refinements based on this continued research. These insights will not only shape the diet's trajectory but also our broader understanding of nutrition and health.

Encouragement for those considering or on their carnivore journey

Taking the step into the carnivore diet can seem daunting, especially given the myriad of dietary choices available today. But for those curious about or already committed to this meat-centric way of life, know that you're not alone. There's a community of supporters, countless success stories, and emerging scientific evidence that can bolster your confidence and resolve.

You're Not Alone

Growing Community: The carnivore diet has garnered a passionate and supportive community. From online forums to local meet-ups, there are countless individuals who share your curiosities and challenges.

Shared Experiences: Hearing stories from others can be both motivating and enlightening. They may share hacks, recipes, or even just words of encouragement that make all the difference on tougher days.

Every Body is Different

Personal Journey: Remember that everyone's experience with the carnivore diet will be unique. Just because one person sees rapid changes doesn't mean everyone will, or should. Be patient and trust your body's pace.

Learning Experience: Every hiccup or challenge can be a learning opportunity. If you encounter cravings or other issues, it's a chance to refine and adjust your approach, making it more sustainable in the long run.

Trust the Process

Adaptation Phase: Like any significant dietary change, the body needs time to adjust. You might face a period of transition where you feel less than optimal, but this is natural. Stick with it, and the benefits can soon follow.

Continuous Growth: As you advance on your journey, you'll grow in knowledge and experience. Each day can offer insights into how different foods affect your mood, energy levels, and overall well-being.

Celebrate Every Victory

Milestones Matter: Whether it's feeling more energetic, losing that first pound, or receiving a positive health report from your doctor, every victory is a testament to your commitment.

Mental Clarity and Well-being: Beyond the physical, the carnivore diet can also bring about positive mental changes. Celebrate the moments of enhanced clarity, focus, or simply feeling good about the choices you're making.

Conclusion

Starting or continuing with the carnivore diet is indeed a courageous decision in today's world of diverse dietary options. But with commitment, support, and a thirst for knowledge, the journey can be profoundly rewarding. Believe in yourself, trust the journey, and know that with every bite, you're taking control of your health in a way that feels right for you.

Share Your Thoughts!

Dear Valued Reader,

Thank you for reading our book about the carnivore diet. This book was created by **Skriuwer**, a group dedicated to providing valuable content that helps people learn and understand more about various topics. Our aim is to offer information that is not only interesting but also thought-provoking, helping you explore the benefits and history of the carnivore diet.

We hope you gained a lot of knowledge about the carnivore diet, its evolution, and why it is becoming popular today. Our goal is to give you insights that help you appreciate the nutritional and health aspects of this diet and how it can impact your lifestyle.

But your involvement doesn't have to stop here. You are a vital part of our community. If you have any comments, questions, or suggestions on how we can improve this book or topics you'd like to see in the future, please email us at **kontakt@skriuwer.com**. Your feedback is very important to us as it helps us create better and more useful content for you and others.

Did you enjoy the book? Please leave a review where you bought it. Your thoughts not only inspire us but also help other readers find and choose this book.

Thank you for choosing **Skriuwer**. Let's continue learning together.

With Appreciation,
The Skriuwer Team

Printed in Great Britain
by Amazon